RESISTANCE BAND EXERCISE MANUAL

Unlock Your Strength, Comprehensive Guide To Mastering Full-Body Fitness, Effective Resistance Band Exercises For Strength, Flexibility, And Mobility

LAMBERT FETTERMAN

DISCLAIMER

The content in this book is offered only for general informative purposes. While every effort has been taken to guarantee the content's accuracy and completeness, the author and publisher accept no responsibility for any mistakes or omissions, or for the results of using the information given herein. The methods, recommendations, and directions in this book are not guaranteed to be appropriate for every person, and readers should exercise caution and seek professional counsel if required before undertaking any of the projects or techniques detailed in this book.

Table of Contents

CHAPTER 1

Introduction To Resistance Bands

Overview Of Resistance Bands

Resistance bands, also known as exercise bands or workout bands, are elastic bands that are flexible and used for strength training, stretching, and rehabilitation. They come in a variety of forms, sizes, and resistance levels, making them suited for people with varying fitness levels and objectives.

Types Of Resistance Bands

Resistance bands are constructed of elastic materials such as rubber or latex and are available in a variety of shapes and sizes, including loop bands, tube bands with handles, and flat bands. They provide variable resistance, which means that when the band is stretched more, the tension rises. Users may change the intensity of their exercises simply by adjusting the length or thickness of the band.

Resistance Bands: There are various varieties of resistance bands, each with its own set of characteristics:

• Loop Bands: These are continuous loops without grips that are used mostly for lower-body workouts such as squats, leg lifts, and lateral walks.

• Tube Bands: These bands feature grips on both ends and are available with or without attachments for a variety of workouts that target different muscle regions.

• Flat Bands: These are narrow, flat bands that are often used for upper body workouts such as arm curls, shoulder presses, and chest flies.

• Figure 8 Bands: These bands, shaped like the number eight, provide particular resistance for workouts like as chest presses and rows.

Benefits Of Using Resistance Bands

1. Resistance bands are versatile in that they may target any muscle group in the body, offering a full-body exercise.

2. They are lightweight and portable, making them ideal for home workouts, travel, and outdoor training.

3. Adjustable Resistance: Bands come in a variety of tension levels, enabling people to grow gradually as they acquire strength.

4. Joint-Friendly: They provide a low-impact choice for people who have joint problems or injuries, allowing for regulated motions and less stress on joints.

5. Resistance bands are an inexpensive fitness tool that may be used for a variety of workouts as compared to other gym equipment.

These bands are designed for those who want to improve their strength, muscular tone, flexibility, and rehabilitation. Resistance bands may be a wonderful addition to your workout regimen, whether you're a novice or an experienced athlete, giving a variety of exercises to challenge and improve your overall fitness level.

CHAPTER 2

Choosing The Right Resistance Band

Finding the correct resistance band is vital for an efficient exercise when it comes to resistance bands. Here is a detailed guide on selecting the appropriate resistance band for your exercise needs:

Understanding Different Resistance Levels

Resistance bands are available in a variety of degrees of resistance, which are often classified by color or resistance level. These bands have variable amounts of tension, making workouts more challenging. Resistance typically varies from mild (yellow or green bands) to heavy (blue or black bands), with some manufacturers using color coding to indicate resistance levels.

• **Light Resistance Bands:** These are appropriate for novices as well as those concentrating on physical therapy and rehabilitation activities. They have the lowest level of stress.

• **Medium Resistance Bands:** These generate moderate tension and are appropriate for intermediate workouts that focus on muscular strength and toning.

• **Heavy Resistance Bands:** These bands are intended for experienced users who want more resistance for muscle growth and strength training.

Selecting The Appropriate Band For Your Fitness Level

The ideal resistance band for you is determined by your fitness objectives, present strength, and the workouts you want to complete. Starting with a mild or medium resistance band is recommended for beginners to become acclimated to the motions without overstretching muscles.

Consider the following elements:

• Fitness Objectives: Determine if you want to tone your muscles, gain strength, or rehab.

• Type of Exercise: Different workouts may need differing degrees of resistance. A hefty resistance band, for example, maybe more suited for lower-body workouts like squats, whilst a softer band may be great for shoulder exercises.

Tips For Purchasing Quality Resistance Bands

Keep the following tips in mind while shopping for resistance bands:

• **Material Quality:** Choose bands made of long-lasting, high-quality latex or rubber. Before making a purchase, look for evidence of rips, warping, or damage.

• **Handles and Attachments:** For added adaptability, some bands include handles or attachments. Check if they are strong and pleasant to handle.

• **Set Variation:** Consider obtaining a set with varying resistance levels to suit different exercises and development in your workouts.

• **Brand Reputation:** Select bands from well-known fitness companies that are recognized for their quality and dependability.

The correct resistance band may be a useful tool for accomplishing your fitness objectives, whether you're wanting to add variation to your training regimen, improve strength, or help in recovery.

CHAPTER 3

Safety Precautions And Warm-Up

When introducing resistance bands into your training program, safety measures and warm-up regimens are essential. Here's a detailed guide:

Importance Of Warming Up Before Using Resistance Bands

A comprehensive warm-up program is required before indulging in any physical activity, including resistance band workouts. It progressively raises heart rate, circulation, and flexibility while lowering the chance of damage.

A dynamic warm-up might consist of modest aerobic exercises such as running or cycling, as well as dynamic stretches to prepare your muscles and joints.

Common Safety Guidelines

1. Before using your resistance bands, always inspect them for wear, tear, or damage. If the band shows indications of wear, such as minor rips or fraying, it should be changed.

2. Anchor Points: Before beginning any activity, make sure the resistance band is properly fastened. The anchoring point should be sturdy and able to resist the band's strain.

3. Start with a level of resistance that enables you to do exercises with good form and technique. As you feel more comfortable and stronger, gradually increase your resistance.

4. Controlled Movements: Carry out workouts with careful, controlled movements. Avoid abrupt or quick movements that might strain muscles or break the band.

5. Maintain a consistent breathing pattern throughout the activity, exhaling during the effort phase and inhaling during the rest period.

6. Correct Form: Maintain good posture and form during each workout. To avoid injury, engage your core and steady your body.

Preparing Your Body For Resistance Band Exercises

1. Warm-up: Start with a few minutes of mild cardiovascular activity, such as jogging or brisk walking, to get your heart rate up and your muscles warmed up.

2. Perform dynamic stretches that simulate the movements you'll be doing throughout your resistance band exercise. These stretches promote flexibility and boost blood flow to the muscles.

3. Include activities that emphasize joint mobility, particularly in regions such as the shoulders, hips, and ankles. This improves the range of motion and gets the joints ready for activity.

4. Activate Muscles: Perform bodyweight exercises or mild motions that engage the muscle areas you'll be targeting before beginning specialized resistance band activities.

You may lessen the risk of injury and enhance the efficiency of your resistance band exercises by following these safety measures and adding a good warm-up program. Always pay attention to your body and discontinue any workout that produces pain or discomfort.

CHAPTER 4

Full-Body Resistance Band Workouts

Resistance bands are an excellent way to exercise various muscle groups while improving strength, flexibility, and endurance. Incorporating these exercises into a full-body workout provides complete muscle activation and improved overall fitness.

Upper Body Exercises

1. Bicep Curls: Stand on the band and grip the handles with your hands facing up. Curls are performed by contracting the biceps and slowly releasing.

2. Step onto the band while gripping the handles at shoulder height. Push the bands aloft while extending your arms, then gently drop them back down.

3. Rowing: Wrap the band around a strong anchor at waist level. Step back and pull the handles towards your body, using the back muscles.

4. Tricep Extensions: Stand on the band while holding one of the handles. Raise your arm upward and stretch your elbow, feeling your triceps engage.

Lower Body Exercises

1. Squats: Stand on the band with your arms at shoulder height. Squat down and return to

a standing posture while keeping resistance in the band.

2. Step onto the band and grip the handles at your sides for lunges. Step back into a lunge, making sure the band provides resistance as you return to the beginning position.

3. **Leg Press:** Sit on the floor with one foot wrapped in the band. Return to a bent-knee posture after extending the leg and pushing against the resistance.

4. Attach the band to a low anchor point for glute kickbacks. Wrap the band around one of your ankles and kick your leg back, activating your glutes.

Core Strengthening Exercises

1. Sit on the floor, wrap the band around your feet, and grasp the handles. Engage the core by twisting the body from side to side.

2. Plank Pulls: Get into a plank posture and pull the band apart, activating the chest and core.

3. Standing Woodchoppers: Using both hands, twist the band handle from high to low across your torso, working the core muscles.

4. Dead Bug: Wrap the band around your feet while holding the grips. Extend the opposing arm and leg while resting on your back, resisting the pull of the band.

By including these exercises in your regimen, you train many muscle groups, resulting in a full-body workout. To optimize results and avoid injury, remember to maintain perfect technique, gradually increase resistance, and allow for enough recovery between sessions.

CHAPTER 5

Targeted Muscle Group Workouts

Resistance bands are versatile and effective at targeting particular muscle areas while fitting a wide range of exercise levels and objectives. Tailoring exercises to specific muscle groups may assist in enhancing outcomes and meeting individual requirements.

Focusing On Specific Muscle Groups

• **Upper Body:** Resistance bands are great for working out the upper body. Bands may be used to do arm exercises such as bicep curls, tricep extensions, and shoulder presses. They efficiently activate muscles by replicating the motion of free weights.

• **Lower Body:** Bands may be used to improve resistance in squats, lunges, leg extensions, and hamstring curls, effectively targeting leg muscles.

• **Core:** Adding bands to workouts such as standing twists, woodchoppers, or sitting rows adds resistance to stimulate core muscles.

• **Back and Chest:** Resistance bands may be used to execute rowing, chest presses, and fly activities, effectively activating muscles in the back and chest.

Customizing Workouts For Different Fitness Goals

• **Strength Training:** Resistance bands may be used to progressively increase resistance levels to gain strength. Adjusting the angle of pull or increasing band tension varies resistance to test muscles and helps in strength increases.

• **Muscle Endurance:** Using lighter bands for more repetitions improves muscle endurance. Circuit-style workouts that include varied activities with short rest periods might improve endurance.

• **Rehabilitation:** By gently exercising muscles and joints, bands offer a safe and regulated way of healing injuries.

They provide resistance without creating undue strain, assisting in the recuperation process.

Combining Exercises For A Comprehensive Routine

• **Full-Body Workouts:** Full-body routines including different resistance band exercises may deliver thorough workouts by engaging several muscle groups. This method guarantees a well-balanced training session.

• **Supersetting and Circuit Training:** Combining workouts in supersets or circuits with little rest times increases the intensity and efficiently activates muscles. Combining upper and lower body workouts, for example, or rotating between various muscle groups in circuits, might increase workout efficiency.

Resistance band exercises may be tailored to particular muscle groups and fitness goals, resulting in a dynamic and complete training regimen that can be adapted to different fitness levels and objectives.

CHAPTER 6

Advanced Resistance Band Techniques

Resistance bands are flexible equipment that may be used for a variety of exercises, making them appropriate for people of all fitness levels. Let's look at some more sophisticated techniques:

Incorporating Progressive Resistance

As your strength grows, it's critical to push your muscles even farther. The process of raising the difficulty of an activity by altering the resistance level is known as progressive resistance. This may be accomplished by utilizing thicker bands, lowering the length of the band, or changing the placement to increase muscular stress.

Using Multiple Bands For Increased Difficulty

Combine different bands to make the task more difficult. This method allows for gradual resistance increases. Looping or piling many bands together may produce significant strain, giving a more demanding exercise for muscle regions that have evolved to lesser resistance levels.

Dynamic Movements And Advanced Exercises

Moving on to dynamic motions tests your stability, balance, and coordination. To work numerous muscular groups at the same time, use exercises such as leaping squats, lateral band walks, and woodchoppers. These motions simulate functional tasks while improving general strength and mobility.

Consider including advanced workouts that target greater muscular groups and core stability, such as resisted push-ups, plank variants, or resistance band deadlifts. These workouts require more muscle activation, which aids in muscular growth and strength development.

To avoid injury, use good form and technique while executing advanced maneuvers. Introduce these activities gradually into your regimen to give your body time to adjust to the additional demands and stress.

Remember that altering your exercises regularly keeps your muscles stimulated and avoids plateaus. Always listen to your body and seek the advice of a fitness expert before progressing to more complicated workouts.

CHAPTER 7

Resistance Band Exercises For Rehabilitation

Individuals undergoing rehabilitation might benefit greatly from resistance band workouts. These exercises provide a diverse and adaptive strategy to gain strength, improve flexibility, and improve general functioning, whether you're healing from an accident or managing chronic diseases. In this part, we'll look at the benefits of resistance band exercises for rehabilitation, detail routines for typical injuries or deficiencies, and talk about working with physical therapists and other healthcare experts.

Rehabilitation Benefits Of Resistance Band Exercises

During the recovery phase, resistance band workouts give a low-impact, regulated technique to improve strength and mobility. Among the many advantages are:

• Progressive Resistance: Resistance bands allow for progressive resistance, which means that resistance may be progressively raised as strength develops. This aspect is critical for those in rehabilitation since it guarantees that the workouts are difficult yet achievable.

• Isolated Muscle Targeting: Resistance bands allow users to isolate certain muscle groups, enabling them to concentrate on strengthening regions impacted by injury or weakness. This method is useful for treating imbalances and fostering healthy muscular growth.

• **Increased Range of Motion:** Many resistance band rehabilitation workouts incorporate controlled, dynamic motions. This aids in the improvement of joint flexibility and range of motion, which is generally a focus in rehabilitation.

• **Versatility:** Resistance bands are available in a variety of resistance levels, making them appropriate for persons at varying stages of recovery. These bands' adaptability allows for a personalized approach to workout routines depending on individual demands and skills.

Exercises For Common Injuries Or Weaknesses

Here are some resistance band workouts that are suited to various frequent ailments or weaknesses:

• External Rotation Exercise for Rotator Cuff Injuries

• Tie the resistance band around your waist.

• Hold the band with the damaged arm while standing perpendicular to the anchor point.

• Maintain a tight grip on the elbow and rotate the arm outward against resistance.

• Leg Press Exercise for Knee Injury

• Attach the resistance band to a strong post at ankle level.

• Sit on the floor, straighten the afflicted leg, and wrap the band around the foot.

• Using the quadriceps, press the leg forward against resistance.

• Cat-Cow Stretch with Band for Lower Back Pain

• Loop the band around the lower back and secure it around a fixed spot.

• Take a tabletop posture on your hands and knees.

• Arch your back upward, straining against the band's resistance, then drop it into a soft curve.

• Dorsiflexion Exercise for Ankle Sprain

• Sit with your legs straight and wrap the band around the ball of your foot.

• Pull the toes towards the body against the band's resistance, concentrating on dorsiflexion.

Working With Physical Therapists And Healthcare Professionals

While resistance band exercises might be useful, a good rehabilitation plan requires collaboration with healthcare specialists, particularly physical therapists. Here's how it's done:

• Individualized plans: Physical therapists may design personalized resistance band workout plans based on the type of injury, current fitness level, and rehabilitation objectives.

• **Progress Monitoring:** Healthcare experts may monitor progress to ensure that the workouts remain demanding but not too stressful. Regular evaluations aid in altering resistance levels and adapting training routines as required.

• **Form and Technique Guidance:** Proper form is critical for the efficacy and safety of resistance band activities. Physical therapists advise patients on proper form and technique to avoid future damage and improve recovery results.

• **Including range:** To avoid boredom and keep the client interested in the rehabilitation process, healthcare practitioners may incorporate a range of resistance band activities. This diversity guarantees that the recuperation process is well-rounded.

Finally, resistance band workouts are a versatile tool for rehabilitation that promotes strength, flexibility, and focused muscle activation. When combined with a complete rehabilitation plan, these activities may considerably aid in the healing process. However, it is critical to collaborate closely with healthcare specialists to ensure that the exercises selected are appropriate for the person and are completed with good form and direction.

CHAPTER 8

Creating Your Own Resistance Band Routine

Resistance band workouts are an adaptable and effective technique to improve strength, flexibility, and general fitness. Several elements must be considered while developing your program to construct a tailored training regimen that meets your demands and objectives.

Designing A Personalized Workout Plan

1. Assessing Fitness Level: To begin, assess your current fitness level. Understanding your skills, shortcomings, and any restrictions is required.

2. **Setting Specific Goals:** Determine your objectives for your resistance band exercises. Having clear objectives leads your exercise, whether it's muscle gain, weight reduction, better flexibility, or rehabilitation.

3. **Exercise Selection:** Select workouts that are in line with your objectives. Resistance bands allow for a variety of motions that target different muscle areas. Include upper and lower body, core, and general functional motions in your workouts.

4. **Balancing Cardio and Strength:** To develop a balanced regimen, use both strength training and cardio routines. This might include switching days or mixing workouts to include both features.

5. Progressive Overload: Gradually increase tension or intensity to keep your muscles challenged. This promotes continuous improvement and avoids plateaus.

6. Consider Rest and Recovery: Schedule rest days into your regimen to give your muscles time to recuperate and repair.

Setting Goals And Tracking Progress

1. Make your objectives as precise as possible. Whether it's the amount of repetitions, sets, or increasing resistance, make it clear what you want to achieve.

2. Quantifiable Objectives: Use quantifiable metrics to track your progress. Maintain a workout log or use an app to track sets,

repetitions, resistance levels, and any changes.

3. **Realistic and Achievable objectives:** Establish realistic objectives that are feasible within a fair period. As you observe modest changes, this keeps you motivated.

4. **Timetable:** Create a timetable for your objectives. This might include short-term objectives in a few weeks and long-term goals spread out over many months.

Adapting Routines For Variety And Continued Motivation

1. Avoid boredom by changing up your workouts, resistance levels, and workout formats. Include a variety of exercises and challenges to keep your practice interesting.

2. Periodization is the division of your routine into periods. For instance, concentrate on endurance in one phase, then strength or power in the next. This minimizes overtraining and promotes well-rounded development.

3. Pay Attention to Your Body's Messages: Pay attention to your body's messages. Adjust the routine if anything seems odd or causes pain. Rest when necessary and avoid pushing through discomfort.

4. Seeking Professional Help: Consult a fitness trainer or physical therapist to create a customized plan suited to your individual goals and limitations.

You may maximize your fitness journey and obtain greater results over time by creating a well-thought-out resistance band training plan, establishing reasonable objectives, and measuring progress.

CHAPTER 9

Nutrition And Recovery For Resistance Band Training

Paying attention to diet and recuperation while introducing resistance band workouts into your regimen may have a big influence on your growth and general well-being. Here's a detailed look at how diet and recovery techniques affect resistance band training:

Importance Of Nutrition In A Resistance Band Workout Plan

1. Workout Fuel: Adequate nourishment gives the energy required for your exercises. Balanced meals that include carbs, proteins,

and healthy fats provide your body with the fuel it needs to do activities successfully.

2. Muscle Repair and Development: Protein consumption is essential for mending muscle tissues and promoting muscular development after resistance band training. Protein-rich diets such as lean meats, beans, dairy, or plant-based protein sources are advised.

3. Staying hydrated is critical for general health and exercise effectiveness. Water contributes to the transfer of nutrients to your muscles and the recuperation process.

Recovery Strategies For Optimal Performance

1. Rest and Sleep: Adequate sleep is essential for healing. Rest allows your muscles to mend and expand. Aim for 7-9 hours of uninterrupted sleep every night.

2. On rest days, include gentle exercise or activities such as yoga, walking, or swimming. It increases blood flow, which aids in muscle repair.

3. Stretching and Mobility Work: Stretching exercises should be performed to promote flexibility and minimize muscular tension. Mobility work promotes joint health and prevents stiffness.

4. Foam rolling and self-massage: Using foam rollers or massage balls to target trigger points helps reduce muscular discomfort and enhance healing.

Tips For Preventing Injuries And Promoting Longevity

1. Proper Form and Technique: Maintain proper form throughout workouts to avoid strain or injury. To guarantee appropriate technique, talk with a trainer or use internet resources.

2. Gradual Progression: To avoid overexertion, allow your body to gradually adjust to greater resistance or intensity levels.

3. Pay alert to any indicators of discomfort or pain in your body. If an activity generates pain that is more than just muscular exhaustion, adjust the action or visit a fitness expert.

4. **Rest Days:** Work rest days into your schedule. Rest is essential for muscle healing and avoiding burnout.

Remember that everyone's dietary requirements and recuperation techniques differ, so it's important to figure out what works best for your body. A nutritionist or fitness expert may give customized advice based on your unique requirements and objectives.

CHAPTER 10

Incorporating Resistance Bands Into Your Lifestyle

Using Resistance Bands At Home, The Gym, Or While Traveling

Resistance bands are very adaptable and portable, making them excellent for a variety of applications. Their versatility is unparalleled, whether at home, the gym, or on the move. Regardless matter where you live, you may add resistance bands into your everyday regimen.

• **At-home exercises:** Use resistance bands at home for full-body exercises. They don't take up much room and provide a variety of workouts that target various muscle areas.

• **Travel-Friendly Fitness:** Bring resistance bands with you when you travel. Because they are lightweight, you can keep up your fitness program wherever you go, guaranteeing continuous workouts even while you are away from home.

• **Gym Complement:** Resistance bands may be used to supplement gym training. They may spice up your workout regimen by providing alternatives to typical weights and equipment.

Encouraging A Consistent Exercise Routine

Any fitness program must be consistent. Resistance band training enables regular exercises since it is simple to use and adaptable to a variety of venues.

• Daily Inclusion: Aim for daily exercises, even if they are brief. Consistency is more important than length; consistency in your program will provide outcomes over time.

• Adaptability to Schedule: Busy schedules may not always allow for a set gym attendance. Having resistance bands on hand allows you to get in brief exercises whenever you have a free minute.

Long-Term Benefits And Sustainability Of Resistance Band Training

Resistance band workouts have several long-term advantages to general health and fitness.

• **Muscular Endurance and Strength:** Consistent resistance band exercises develop muscular endurance and strength over time, resulting in better posture and a lower chance of injury.

• **Functional Fitness:** Resistance bands increase functional strength, which transfers into everyday motions, making them simpler and lowering the risk of strains or aches.

• Joint Health and Flexibility: The regulated resistance provided by bands promotes joint health and flexibility, which is necessary for general mobility and injury prevention.

Convenience And Sustainability

One of the most notable benefits of resistance bands is their long-term use in fitness programs.

• Low-Cost and Long-Term Use: Unlike pricey gym memberships or cumbersome workout equipment, resistance bands are low-cost, long-term use.

• Family and Group exercises: They may be used for both family and group exercises.

You may promote communal fitness objectives by sharing the advantages of resistance band exercise with friends and family.

• **Changing Workouts:** Resistance bands allow for advancement. You can effortlessly modify the resistance as your fitness level increases, assuring continual challenge and improvement.

Incorporating resistance bands into your lifestyle is an adaptable, accessible, and long-term approach to general well-being.

Conclusion

Finally, resistance band exercises provide a varied and effective method of strength training that is appropriate for people of all fitness levels and objectives. Throughout this guide, we've covered everything you need to know about incorporating resistance bands into your exercise regimen, from choosing the correct bands to safety measures and warm-up methods to focused muscle group workouts and advanced techniques.

It has been underlined the value of resistance bands in rehabilitation and building a specific training regimen suited to your requirements and objectives. In addition, we investigated the effect of diet and recuperation on resistance band training performance, injury prevention, and lifespan.

We investigated the adaptation of resistance bands to various lifestyles, whether used at home, in the gym, or when traveling, to establish a regular workout habit for long-term benefits. Individuals may attain long-term fitness and well-being by adopting a holistic approach that blends resistance band workouts with an adequate diet, recovery measures, and a dedication to consistency.

Remember that resistance bands are not only accessible and inexpensive, but they also add to overall strength, flexibility, and functional fitness. Accept the adaptability and ease that resistance band workouts provide as you adopt them into your lifestyle, making fitness a fun and sustainable part of your everyday regimen.

Resistance band exercises, in essence, are more than just workouts; they are a way of life that promotes health, energy, and a feeling of well-being. You are well-equipped to begin on a path of increased strength, resilience, and lifetime fitness with the information and techniques presented in this course.

THE END